# Beyond

## 50

### *Shades...*

## A Guide for
## Healthy Sexual Communication

By Na'Im Ansar Najieb

# DEDICATION

## This Guide is Dedicated to
## YOU

**Thank You**

# ABOUT THE EDUCATIONAL GUIDES SERIES

Welcome to another educational Guide by
*Love 101!*

*What is the Purpose of these Guides?*

The Purpose of these Guides is to support your efforts
To create and maintain Healthy Relationships.

*How do the Guides support you?*

By offering clarity and equipping you with
Practical tools to use and apply regarding the topic at hand.

*What is the series about?*

This Guide on *Healthy Sexual Communication* is part of
A series of Guides that address many topics of life and relationships

---

## THESE TOPICS INCLUDE

| | | |
|---|---|---|
| *Sexuality* | *Living With People* | *Romance* |
| *Socializing* | *Dating* | *Long Distance* |
| *Networking* | *Family Dynamics* | *And Much More!* |

---

## FOR MORE INFORMATION

| | |
|---|---|
| *Visit* | Contact |
| NaimNajieb.com | Naim@NaimNajieb.com |

---

Now, Prepare to enjoy:

## Beyond 50 Shades...: *A Guide For Healthy Sexual Communication*

*Love 101 Publications*
Copyright © 2020

# Table Of Contents


Sexual Communication Assessment     5
Results     6
Is This Guide For You?     7
Introduction     8


# PART I
## MINDSEX     10
### *What Is Your <u>Mindset</u> Around Sex?*


**Chapter 1: SETTING THE GOAL**     6

**Chapter 2: NEEDS VS DESIRES**     13
    *How to Approach Needs & Desires*     22
    *Love Yourself First*     24
    *Practice Rephrasing*     25

**Chapter 3: HOLDING SPACE**     28
    *Responsibilities*     31
    **Giver and Receiver**     32
      ***<u>Responsibilities of the Giver</u>***     33
      ***<u>Responsibilities of the Receiver</u>***     35
    *The Importance of Practicing Holding Space*     36
    *Making A Request For Space To Be Held For You*     38
    *Practice Requesting*     40

**Chapter 4: CREATING A SAFE SPACE**     42
    *Finding Your Totem*     45
    *<u>Safe Space Rules</u>*     47
    *Appreciate Each Other*     48
    **Appreciation Exercise**     49
    **Cheat Codes:** *What Is A Safe Space For?*     51


# PART II
## SEXPLORATION     52
### *What Is Your <u>Mindset</u> Around Sex?*


**Chapter 5: SEX?**     54
    **Conversation Questions:** *About Sex*     55

# Table Of Contents
### Continued...


**Chapter 6: SEXUAL HEALTH?**     57
Conversation Questions: *Sexual Health*     58

**Chapter 7: SEXUAL IDENTITY?**     61
Conversation Questions: *Sexual Identity*     62

**Chapter 8: SEXUAL EXCLUSIVITY?**     63
Conversation Questions: *Sexual Exclusivity*     67

**Chapter 9: CONSENT?**     69
Conversation Questions: *Clarifying Consent*     73
*Consent Is Not Always Verbal*     74
Chart: *Creating Consent Symbols*     75

**Chapter 10: FOREPLAY?**     77
Conversation Questions: *Foreplay*     79

**Chapter 11: TURN ON AND TURN OFFS?**     80
*Communicating About Turn Ons and Turn Offs*     81
Conversation Questions     81
Cheat Codes Chart: *Turn Ons and Turn Offs*     82

**Chapter 12: KINKS AND FETISHES?**     84
Kinky Conversation Exploration Guide     88

**Chapter 13: PORN?**     94
Conversation Questions:     95

**Chapter 14: EROTIC JOURNAL?**     96
Cheat Codes: *Erotic Journal*     97
Starting Your Erotic Journal Together     98
*Erotic Journal Entry Guide*     98

**ABOUT THE AUTHOR**     101
**CONTACT INFORMATION**     102

# SEXUAL COMMUNICATION ASSESSMENT

### *Determining Your Sexual Comfort Level*

Answer the following questions with a simple "yes" or "no" answer.

*If you watch porn, do you ever watch it with your Partner?*
*(Y / N)*

*Have you shared your sexual fantasies with your Partner?*
*(Y / N)*

*Have you talked to your Partner about their turn ons and turn offs?*
*(Y / N)*

*Have you talked to your Partner about YOUR turn ons and turn offs?*
*(Y / N)*

*During or after sex,*
*Do you tell your Partner what they did that you especially enjoyed?*
*(Y / N)*

*Do you ask them what they enjoy about your sexual interplay?*
*(Y / N)*

*Have you discussed the topic of sexual exclusivity or nonexclusivity*
*In your relationship lately?*
*(Y / N)*

*Are you and your Partner(s) on the same page about sexual exclusivity?*
*(Y / N)*

***Do you feel safe to talk to your Partner about anything***
***Regarding sex and sexuality?***
***(Y / N)***

***Is your level of ease in communicating about sexuality with your Partner***
***Improving everyday?***
***(Y / N)***

***Do you and your Partner educate yourselves about sexuality?***
***I.e. read books, go to classes,***
***And/or watch educational content about sexuality?***
***(Y / N)***

## SCORING

For every **"yes"** answer, give yourself *1 point.*

For every **"no"** answer, subtract *-1 point.*

Any answer that you're not sure about is a "no".

## RESULTS

If you scored less than 10 (100%), you need this Guide in your life.
Grab your Partner and start reading with them ***right now.***

And even if you scored a 10,
You might still learn a thing or two.

***Ready to learn?***

**Let's begin.**

# IS THIS GUIDE FOR YOU?

### *Answer These Questions Before Continuing*

*Are you in a sexually active relationship or considering
Becoming sexually active in your relationship?*

*Do you have sexual fantasies that you want to explore?*

*Do you feel there is something blocking you from
Freely and fully expressing yourself sexually?*

*Do you want to be able to share what's on your mind about
Sex without fear?*

*Do you want to explore your turn ons and wildest fantasies?*

*Do you want to know what turns your Partner on sexually?*

*Do you want to know how sexually compatible
You and your Partner are?*

*If you are in a sexual relationship,
Would you like to deepen the sexual connection?*

---

*If you answered "yes" to any of these questions…*

**Good news!**

This Guide is for you.

*Please use responsibly.*

# INTRODUCTION
## *Some Things to Think About*

*When is the last time you used a conversation to*
*Explore your sexuality?*

*When is the last time you had an open adult conversation*
*With your sexual Partner about sex?*

This Guide is written from the following standpoint:

## <u>SEXUAL COMMUNICATION</u>
*Sexual communication should be refreshing,*
*And should flow like fresh running water*

Unfortunately, sex and sexuality is simultaneously
One of the **most desired and most taboo** topics
Of conversation and exploration.

### *Why?*

Because like most people, you've been scarred by
Fear-based cultural and religious beliefs and teachings.

These teachings shroud the topic of sexuality
In guilt, shame, ignorance and fear.

### NO MORE!

*How would you like to talk about sex as easily*
*As you talk about the weather?*

*How would you like to save yourself years of sexual frustration
Ignorance and confusion?*

*How would you like to explore both you and your Partner's
Sexual desires in a safe, judgment-free zone?*

*How would you like to learn how to create an environment
Where you can openly express your deepest darkest fantasies?*

If so,
You're in the right place.

*Ready to communicate?*

*Cum on...*

**Let's do it!**

# Part I

# MINDSEX

## *What Is Your <u>Mindset</u> Around Sex?*

Welcome to Part I of this Guide!

This Guide consists of two Parts.
Each part will equip you with different tools to support
Healthy sexual communication in your relationship.

Here is an important thing to note about this Guide…

## THIS IS AN INTERACTIVE GUIDE!!!

*This is not just a book you read, this is a book you DO...*
*With your Partner.*

Throughout this Guide there will be activities to do
and conversations to have.

*Let's take a snapshot of the first Part...*
*(The Part you are reading now)*

In this first Part,
You will learn the mental and emotional tools required for
Healthy sexual communication.

*In other words…*

**Adopting a healthy mindset.**

A healthy mindset around sex is needed to strengthen
The connection between you and your Partner.

And as you well know…

*Sex starts in the mind.*

---

## SEXUAL CONNECTION PRINCIPLE
### *Sex Is A Mental Activity Before It Is A Physical Activity*

---

In Part I you will learn the following:

- **Setting the Goal**
  - *Deciding the purpose for your sexual exploration*

- **The difference between desires and needs**
  - *Why it is dangerous to confuse the two*

- **How to hold a loving space for each other**
  - *Creating an emotional clearing for stuff to come up*

- **How to create a safe space for each other**
  - *Creating a judgment free-zone to express yourselves freely in your relationship*

- **An Appreciation exercise**
  - *Deepening your connection with appreciation*

### In Part II
You will start on your actual "Sexploration" together.
Here, you will explore many sexual communication topics.

*How will you explore these topics?*

**Through conversation!**

You will have specific conversations that will help you learn more
About your Partner and more about yourself.

The purpose of these conversations is to deepen your connection
And save you time by asking important questions.

**These topics and conversations include:**

- **Sex and Sexuality**
- **Sexual Identity**
- **Sexual Health**
- **Sexual Exclusivity**
- **Consent**
- **Foreplay**
- **Turn ons & turn offs**
- **Kinks and fetishes**
- **Porn**
- **Starting a erotic/sexual journal**

*Fun topics right?!*

Before we get into that,
Let's get your mind right.

*Ready for your mindsex training?*

**Let's begin!**

# Chapter 1
# SETTING THE GOAL
### *What's The Purpose?*

*"Why are we having sex anyway? "*
*"Why do we want to have sex with each other?"*

***Have you asked each other these questions lately?***

They are good questions to ask.

Because if all you can come up with is…

***"I'm horny…And you're right there…Sooo…"***

This Guide is going to push you to go a little further than that.

### <u>TRUTH PRINCIPLE</u>
***Bodies Cannot Join And Become One***
***Minds Can Join and Become One***

**Sex starts in the mind.**

*Remember the Purpose of this Guide?*

This is a Guide for Healthy Sexual Communication.

*And where does communication start?*

**Communication starts in the mind.**

You are currently reading the first part of this Guide
Which deals exclusively with the mind.

We'll get to the physical stuff in Part II.

Before we get to that physical connection,
You and your Partner must have a strong mental connection.

You've been taught ass-backwards.

You've been taught to have sex with someone *as a way*
To feel connected to them.

That's the lie.

*Here's the Truth:*

### <u>THE TRUTH</u>
***You should feel connected to each other***
***Long before you ever have sex***

In this way, when you do have the sex,
It will be outstanding!

**"So how do we create this mental connection?"**

It start with this:

**SETTING THE GOAL**

*What is setting the goal?*

Setting the goal is about being on the same page
About why you're in a sexual relationship with each other.

*"How do we set the goal?"*

Easy…

Have a conversation.

## SETTING THE GOAL
## CONVERSATION QUESTIONS
*Ask These Questions to Each Other*

*What is the purpose of our relationship?*

*Why are we together?*

*What is the purpose of having sex in our relationship?*

*Why are we having sex with each other?*

*What do we want to experience by having sex?*

*What higher purpose do we want our sex to serve?*

*Why are we reading this book together?*

*What do we want to gain by reading this book?*

***Have this conversation now***

*So…*
*What did you learn?*

*Are you more clear about your relationship now?*

*Did you realize that all of those question are really*
*The same question, asked in a different form?*

Your answer to every questions could literally be:

**"To have fun and deepen our loving connection"**

**EXAMPLE**
*What is the purpose of our relationship?*
**"To have fun and deepen our loving connection"**

*What is the purpose of having sex in our relationship?*
**"To have fun and deepen our loving connection"**

*Why are we having sex with each other?*
**"To have fun and deepen our loving connection"**

*What do we want to experience by having sex?*
**"To have fun and deepen our loving connection"**

*Make sense?*

This is a conversation you can revisit at any time.

You can never be too clear about why you are
Joining your life with another person.

When you have established a purpose for your relationship
And for your sex, you are on the same page mentally.

**You are connected. You are clear. You are on purpose.**

So you never have to wonder about why you're together.

And if you ever get confused or forgetful,
Have the conversation again.

**Refocus.**

*Moving on.*

In the next chapter, we are going to discuss a very basic,
Very simple, and very *overlooked* topic.

The confusion that surrounds this topic
Causes major miscommunication and separation.

*What's the topic?*

The topic is:

***Needs VS Desires***

Let's go back to basics.

# Chapter 2

# NEEDS VS DESIRES

*Survival vs Wants...There's A BIG Difference*

You've probably heard the phrase:

*"Getting your needs met" or "Meeting your needs".*

We're going to explore the difference between
Needs and desires in this chapter.

There is a lot of confusion and dangerous misinformation
Around this topic.

Most relationship Guides and experts will tell you
That for your relationship to be healthy you have to:

*"Communicate your needs"*
*"Listen to your Partner's needs"*
*"Compromise so you can get your needs met"*

**NO.**

None of that is true.
This is a misunderstanding that is detrimental
To any healthy relationship.

*Why?*

Because of this Principle for healthy Relationships:

---

### <u>HEALTHY RELATIONSHIP PRINCIPLE</u>
*Healthy Relationships Are <u>NOT</u> A Place to Get Your Needs Met*

---

Relying on a relationship and another person
To get your needs met puts undue strain on the relationship.

It also makes you come across as needy.
Not to mention, being needy is *HIGHLY UNATTRACTIVE*.

*What do we mean by "needs"?*

Let's define it:

---

## "NEEDS" DEFINITION
### *Anything Required for Your Survival*

---

## "NEEDS" INCLUDE

- Food
- Clothing
- Water
- Transportation
- Security/Safety

- Clean Air
- Healthcare
- Money
- Facilities
- Lodging

---

## "NEEDS" PRINCIPLE
### *Everyone's Needs Are Exactly The Same*
### *Everyone Requires The Same Basic Needs for Survival*

---

*As an adult, guess who is responsible for meeting your needs?*

**YOU ARE!**
**NO ONE ELSE!**

*And guess who is responsible for meeting the needs of others?*

**THEY ARE!**
**NOT YOU!**

# <u>"NEEDS" PRINCIPLE</u>
*You Are Responsible for Meeting Your Own Needs*
*You Are NOT Responsible for Meeting Anyone Else's Needs*

*So why are so many sources teaching that it is appropriate to*
*Make your needs your Partner's responsibility?*

Because they are not really talking about needs at all.

*What are they talking about?*

**They are talking about *DESIRES*.**

*In other words "wants".*

Let's take a look at some common desires.
*In other words…*

## <u>NOT NEEDS</u>
*You do not need the following to survive*

- Sex
- Romance
- A relationship
- To get married
- Your feelings to be validated
- Your Partner to listen to how you feel
- Your Partner to understand how you feel
- Your Partner to take care of you
- To be in constant contact with your Partner
- To know where your Partner is
- To receive a text back when you text
- To receive a call back when you call

Not receiving any of those things won't kill you.

---

# "DESIRES" PRINCIPLE
*You Are Responsible for Meeting Your Own Desires*
*You Are NOT Responsible for Meeting Anyone Else's Desires*

---

**It is EXTREMELY DANGEROUS to your relationship
To confuse needs and desires.**

*Why is it dangerous to confuse needs and desires?*

Because it causes communication breakdown in the relationship.

*How does communication breakdown occur?*

When someone says:

*"I NEED you to listen to me right now!"*

They are using the WORD "need" incorrectly in that statement.
What they are really talking about is what they *desire.*

*How do you know?*

Ask yourself:

*"Will they die if I don't listen to them right now?"*
*"Will they die if I don't listen to them at all?"*

**No. They won't die.**

*Therefore,*
Listening to what someone wants to say to you is not a need.

Check out the following Cheat Codes Chart for clarity on how Desires are usually expressed as needs.

| CHEAT CODES CHART FOR CLARIFYING NEEDS AND DESIRES | |
| --- | --- |
| **WHAT IS SAID** | **WHAT IS MEANT** |
| I have sexual needs | I have sexual desires |
| I have emotional needs | I have emotional desires |
| I need you to hear me right now<br>I need to be heard | I want you to hear what I have to say right now<br>I want to be heard by you |
| I need sexual exclusivity | I desire sexual exclusivity |
| I need you to hold me | I want you to hold me |
| I need you | I desire you |
| I need some space<br>I need to be alone | I desire some space<br>I want to be alone |
| I need to know what's bothering you | I want to know what's bothering you |

*Clear?*

*So how can you tell if something is a need vs a desire?*

DISTINGUISHING "NEEDS" VS "DESIRES
*Ask Yourself:*
*"Will I die if I don't get this?"*

If the answer is:
*"No, I won't die if I don't get this"*

**Then you are certainly talking about a desire, not a need.**

It's that simple.

**Moving on.**

*Let's talk about...*

# HOW TO APPROACH NEEDS AND DESIRES
*Take Responsibility*

Do not place your needs on any other person.
It is not their responsibility to take care of you.

Don't receive any relationship where someone tries
To make you responsible for their needs.

**You are their Partner not their parent.**

Also, do not accept guilt-trips or ultimatums from
People who are disappointed when you
Don't do what they want you to do.

**PEOPLE WHO SAY...**

*"You don't care about me..."*
*"I'm so upset with you..."*
*"If you don't...[do this thing]...I'm not talking to you."*

**Too bad.**

**You may say:**

*"I know I don't need sex to survive,*
*But I need it to have a happy and fulfilled life."*

**NOT TRUE.**

## <u>HAPPINESS AND FULFILLMENT PRINCIPLE</u>
*No One Can "Make" You Happy or Fulfilled*
*You Are Responsible for Your Own Happiness and Fulfillment*

Do not attach your basic survival needs,
Or your personal desires and preferences to anyone else.

That is a recipe for calamity.

*"What about desires?*
*Aren't we in a relationship to bring each other pleasure?"*

The purpose of your relationship is whatever you both decide it is.

Even if you decide that you are together
To bring each other pleasure,
You will not be able to pull it off in every situation every time.

**It is simply not possible.**

Review the "Happiness and Fulfillment Principle".

**It is your responsibility.**

The bottom line is this...

*No one is responsible for fulfilling your desires.*
*And you are not responsible for fulfilling their desires.*

Everything you give each other is a gift!

*For example...*

Let's say you enjoy receiving massages from your Partner.

**YOU**
*Can you give me a massage?*

**PARTNER**
*I don't want to right now.*

**QUESTION**
*Can you file charges against them and bring them to court*
*For not giving you a massage?*

**No.**

You can try. And you will be laughed out of the courthouse.

*That said,*
Let's conclude this chapter with this message...

# LOVE YOURSELF FIRST
### *Take Care of Your Needs First*

You have survival needs.
You are responsible for meeting your needs.

No person is responsible for meeting any of your needs
At any time.

When you join in a relationship,
Join as a whole person who takes care of all of their own needs.
And join others who also take care of all of their own needs.

In this way, you can enjoy your relationships without
The strain of anyone's needs depending on it.

# PRACTICE REPHRASING
## *You Don't <u>Need</u> to Say "Need"*

To drive this lesson home, you need to practice.

Here is a simple exercise you can start doing right now,
With or without a Partner.

### PURPOSE OF THIS EXERCISE

The purpose of this exercise is to bring more awareness
To how often you (and others) use the word "need".

The purpose is also to correct yourself when you are
Using the word "need" incorrectly.

*Meaning…*

When you are saying "need"
But really referring to something you want/desire.

See how it's done in the next section

# HOW IT'S DONE
### *Stop Saying "Need"*

Whenever you catch yourself saying *"I need…"* to someone,
**STOP!**
And rephrase what you're saying as:


*"I want…"* **or** *"I would like…"*


Check out the examples in the Cheat Codes Chart below.

| EXAMPLES OF REPHRASING "NEEDS" TO "WANTS" | |
|---|---|
| **WHAT YOU MAY SAY/ASK** | **HOW YOU CAN REPHRASE** |
| *"I need to see you"* | *"I would like to see you"* |
| *"I need a napkin please"* | *"I would like a napkin please"* |
| *"I need you to talk to me"* <br> *"We need to talk"* | *"I would like you to talk to me"* <br> *"I would like for us to talk"* |
| *"What do you need me to do?"* | *"What do you want me to do?"* |
| *"What do you need?"* | *"What do you want?"* |
| *"I need you"* | *"I want you"* / *"I desire you"* |

When you start doing this exercise,
You'll quickly become aware of how inappropriately
The word "need" is applied to non-survival-based things.

Your job here is not to correct anybody,
Especially if they are not doing this exercise with you.


Your job is simply to become aware of how YOU
Are using the word "need" and rephrase properly.
Especially when speaking with others.


This is an ongoing practice that is aimed at deprogramming
Your misconceptions about desires vs. needs.


***How will practicing this help you deprogram?***


By actively checking yourself when you speak.


You will begin seeing needs and desires more clearly,
And your communication with *everyone*
In your life will greatly benefit.

---


Now let's talk about something that is vital not only to
To your healthy *sexual* communication,
And your healthy communication in general.

# Chapter 3
# HOLDING SPACE
*Creating A Loving Clearing*

In order to have healthy sexual communication,
There are some important skills you must develop.

The skill we will talk about in this chapter is called:
**"Holding space", or "Creating a Clearing".**

This is a skill you absolutely must learn how to use
If you want to have deep sexual communication
And connection with your Partner.

*So what does it mean to hold space for someone?*

It means to be the presence of empathy and compassion
For someone during their most vulnerable moments.

Just like preparing a room (physical space) for someone to rest in,
Holding space does the same thing on an emotional level.
It is the decision to create an emotional safe zone
For them to be vulnerable in.

*What is the Purpose of Holding Space for someone?*

The purpose is to allow healing to occur in whatever way
It needs to for them, and for you both.
And healing can only occur when the
Emotional environment is safe.

*What does holding space for my Partner look like?*

It could look like anything...

*It may be listening while they express*
*Something that is on their heart.*

*It may be giving them physical space when they want to be alone.*

*It may be just holding them.*

It's not important what happens when you're holding space.
What's important is that you are doing the healing work together.

---

## HOLDING SPACE
*Holding Space Is About A Heart-Space (Emotional Space)*
*Not A Head-Space (Mental Space)*
*Not A Location (Physical Space)*

---

In the next chapter we will cover how to create a "safe space"
For your communication to occur.

Right now,
We are going to discuss the two most important things
Required of you and your Partner when it comes
To "holding space" for each other.

*What are these two important things?*

1. **Mindset**
   a. *Your mindset when holding space*
   b. *Your mindset when having space held for you*

2. **Responsibilities**
   a. *Your responsibilities when holding space*
   b. *Your responsibilities when having space held for you*

# MINDSET
## *For Holding Space*

*What should be your mindset when you are
Holding space for your Partner?*

**Your mindset should be open and loving.**

Here are some thoughts that should be going through your mind
When you are holding space for your Partner

## YOUR MINDSET WHEN HOLDING SPACE

*"I'm here for you"*      *"I am here to help"*
*"I support you"*      *"I want what's best for you"*
*"I hear you"*      *"We are the same"*
*"I care about you"*      *"I will not attack you"*
*"I relate to you"*      *"You're safe"*
*"We're on the same team"*      *"I appreciate you"*
*"You're Innocent"*      *"I Trust you"*
*"You haven't done anything wrong"*
*"Whatever you share or don't share is ok with me"*

These are the thoughts you should be thinking.
You do not necessarily have to say them out loud,
Unless it is helpful to do so.

---

*What if I am the one requesting my Partner to hold space for me?
What should my mindset be?*

If you are asking your Partner to hold space for you
And they agree, your mindset should also be open.

You should allow whatever feelings inside of you to come up,
And remember that you are supported and loved no matter what.

## MINDSET WHEN RECEIVING SPACE
## BEING HELD FOR YOU

*"I am loved"*               *"I will not be attacked"*
*"I am safe"*                 *"I am open"*
*"I am supported"*          *"I can take my time"*
*"I am cared for"*          *"I am Innocent"*
*"I am appreciated"*       *"I am fully heard"*
*"We're on the same team"*   *"Whatever comes up is ok"*
*"We are the same"*          *"I Trust my Partner"*
*"I haven't done anything wrong"*
*"Whatever I share or don't share is ok"*

# RESPONSIBILITIES
*For Holding Space*

Holding space is not meant to be used as an
Ongoing therapy session about the same issues.

It's meant to be an opportunity for you as Partners to heal through
Sexual and communication blocks together.

This means there are specific responsibilities you both must
Understand and commit to before you even request
Or choose to hold space for one another.

***What are the responsibilities?***

There are 2 sets of responsibilities for the 2 roles that are played…

# GIVER AND RECEIVER
## *Responsibilities*

1. Your responsibilities in the role of holding space/creating the clearing for your Partner
   a. *We will call this role: "The Giver"*

2. Your responsibilities in the role of receiving your Partner holding space/creating a clearing for you
   a. *We will call this role: "The Receiver"*

## RESPONSIBILITIES OF <u>THE GIVER</u>

Your responsibility as the Giver is to be the **NURTURER**
In that moment/session.

### *What does that mean?*

That means you have an important decision to make
Before you say:

### *"Yes, I will hold space/create a clearing for you"*

### *What decision do you have to make?*

You have to make a decision to embrace ALL of the
Responsibilities of being the Giver while holding space
For your Partner.

### *What are those responsibilities?*

[See responsibilities of the Giver on next page]

# RESPONSIBILITIES OF THE GIVER

- I will maintain a positive, loving, nurturing energy towards my Partner
- I will make this moment *all about them* and what's on their heart, not about me
  - *I am here only to witness them and provide comfort if requested*
- I will not take anything my Partner says personally
- I will not take anything that comes up for my Partner personally
- I will not make their moment of vulnerability about me
- I will not try to fix them
- I will not allow them to use this moment to attack me or our relationship
- I will not allow them to use this moment to attack themselves
- I will reassure them that I am here for them
- I will be patient with them
- I will not try to rush them or force anything out of them
- I will not be attached to a specific form of outcome from this session
- I will let them know if I no longer feel I have the capacity to hold space for them in any moment
- I will judge nothing that occurs
- I will expect nothing in return for doing this
- I will respect my Partner and their boundaries at all times
- I will be fully present with my Partner at all times

---

Those are your responsibilities as the Giver.
Meaning, if you are going to hold space for your Partner.

*[Bookmark this page!]*

## REMEMBER YOUR FREEDOM!

*If it feels like too much at any time to hold space...*

## DO NOT HOLD SPACE FOR THEM AT THE TIME

*Simple.*

It takes an energetic commitment to make a moment
**ENTIRELY** about someone else.

And it is understandable if you
*Simply don't have it in you at the time.*

Or you simply don't want to.

Don't write the check if you feel
Your emotional bank account is depleted.

You will only hurt yourself and resent your Partner.

*And resentment causes separation,
Not communication.*

## REMEMBER YOUR PURPOSE
*Your purpose for doing this healing work is to create
A deeper connection with your Partner*

*Therefore,*
If you're doing something (even talking or "holding space")
And you feel disconnected while you're doing it...

## STOP DOING IT!
## JUST STOP!

Now, it's time to look at your responsibilities as the Receiver.

# **<u>RESPONSIBILITIES OF THE RECEIVER</u>**

- I will take total responsibility for what I am feeling at this moment
- I will allow whatever is coming up for me in this moment to be healed and released
- I will share what's on my heart without censoring myself
- I will not make what I'm feeling or going through about my Partner
- I will allow myself to be vulnerable
- I will remember that there is nothing wrong with me for having an emotional experience
- I will not attack my Partner for any reason
- I will not attack myself for any reason
- I will be patient with myself
- I will not rush myself
- I will not be attached to a specific form of outcome from this session
- I will allow myself to stop sharing at any time and know that it is ok
- I will not judge myself
- I will thank my Partner for being there for me at this time
    - *I will express appreciation because they do not owe me their time or energy*
    - *I will not waste their time or mine*
- I will allow whatever block coming up to be fully released
    - *I do not intend to talk or vent about the same things over and over again*
- I will respect my Partner & their boundaries at all times
- I will remain fully present with my Partner at all times

*[Bookmark this page!]*

You should read these responsibilities aloud to each other
*Before deciding to hold space.*

**The responsibilities of the Giver and the Receiver
Can be summed up as follows:**

## <u>RESPONSIBILITIES SUMMARY</u>

*The Giver is responsible to devote the present moment
ENTIRELY to the Receiver
The Receiver is responsible TO DO THEIR VERY BEST
To heal (release their blocks) in that moment*

# THE IMPORTANCE OF PRACTICING HOLDING SPACE
### *Mutually and Consensually*

Holding space for one another is a powerful tool
For practicing healthy communication and openness.
Be it about sex or anything at all.

It requires Trust and acceptance of yourself and your Partner.

It is an exercise in mindfulness and appreciation.
Appreciation and mindfulness about the time and energy
That your Partner is sharing with you.

Everyone has held space for someone at some point.
*Usually multiple times a day.*

The problem is,
Most people will demand your time and energy nonconsensually.

And they are usually unaware of the energetic strain
The exchange is placing on you.

Those are not fair exchanges,
And you will end up energetically drained.

We call those kinds of exchanges *"emotional drive-bys"*,
And those kinds of people *"energy vampires"*.

*How do you know if you're dealing with an energy vampire?*

**Here are some signs you're dealing with an energy vampire...**

# IDENTIFYING ENERGY VAMPIRES
## *What Are Their Character Traits?*

- Energy vampires complain complain complain
- Energy vampires dump their problems and drama on you without consent or warning
- Energy vampires make the interaction all about them
- Energy vampires expect you to be their sounding board
- Energy vampires talk about the same issues, the same people, and the same problems over and over again
- Energy vampires are pretty consistent energy vampires
  - *They behave this way with many people in their lives, not just you*

**So how do you make sure YOU don't behave**
**As an energy vampire?**

**Here's how...**

# MAKING A REQUEST TO HOLD SPACE FOR YOU

*"Will You Create A Clearing for Me In This Moment?"*

**First things first…**

*What does it ultimately mean when you request
For your Partner to hold space for you?*

---

### REQUESTING TO HOLD SPACE

*Asking your Partner's CONSENT to offer their time and energy
To make the moment ENTIRELY about you*

---

*When do you request your Partner to hold space for you?*

- When you feel you have something on your heart to share
- When a block comes up and you want your Partner's help in releasing it
- When you want your Partner's emotional support and undivided attention

*"How do I know what to say, ask or share
When I am requesting my Partner to hold space?"*

There are a couple of questions you can ask yourself that
Will help you communicate what's truly on your heart.

Ask yourself these questions when opening up
And expressing yourself to your Partner.

*[See "The Heart of the Matter" on next page]*

# <u>THE HEART OF THE MATTER</u>

*What Would I Say to You if I Knew*
*I Wouldn't be Attacked for Saying it?*

*What Would I Ask You if I Knew*
*I Wouldn't be Attacked for Asking it?*

## EXAMPLE OF REQUESTING PARTNER TO HOLD SPACE

*"I have something I want to share with you,*
*And I would like for you to listen.*
*Will you hold space for me in this moment?"*

## REMEMBER YOUR RESPONSIBILITY
## TO YOUR PARTNER!

If they say:

*"Yes, I will hold space for you..."*

That does not mean you can use this as an opportunity to:

- *Attack them*
- *Guilt trip them*
- *Try to change them*
- *Close down to them*

Your emotional issues are your own.
They have nothing to do with your Partner.

They are being gracious by gifting you their time, energy,
Undivided attention and empathy.

**You are not entitled to any of those things from them.**

The least you can do is offer them your willingness
To make an effort to release and get over
Whatever is troubling you.

Do not assume that just because they are your Partner
And they are in a relationship with you that they owe you
Their time and energy.

**They don't.**
**They just don't.**

And you don't owe anyone your time and energy either.

Now let's practice.

# PRACTICE REQUESTING
*Every Time*

Here's a good practice you can do to remind yourselves of
Your responsibilities while holding space.

### PARTNER 1
*I'm feeling disconnected and separate from you right now.*
*Are you willing to create a clearing for me in this moment?*

### PARTNER 2
*Are you willing to take responsibility for how you feel in this moment*
*And do your best to release any disconnected and separate feelings?*

### PARTNER 1
*Yes I am*

**PARTNER 2**

[Smiles]

*Yes, I will create a clearing for you…*
*Let's set up our safe space so we can talk.*

---

That leads us directly to our next topic of discussion...

*What is a safe space?*

*What does a safe space entail?*

*How do you create a safe space?*

**Turn the page to find out.**

# Chapter 4

# CREATING A SAFE SPACE

## *Making It Safe To Communicate*

### SCENARIO

Two Partners are together in a private setting.

Partner 1 pulls out a small rug and lays it out on the floor.
Partner 2 brings a bowl of fruit and places it in the middle
Of the rug.

They both sit down facing each other.

### PARTNER 1

*Are you ready?*

### PARTNER 2

*Yes, are you?*

### PARTNER 1

*Yes.*

*[Partner 2 feeds a grape to Partner 1]*

### PARTNER 2

*So...Have you ever tried anal?*

[Pause]

---

***What happened here? What was that?***
That was an example of two people creating a safe space
To communicate about their sexuality.

Everything they did had a meaning to them and
Was for the purpose of feeling safe.

Before you can casually and freely discuss the topic of sex,
There is some work you have to do that will NOT feel
Casual or natural.

**And it starts with creating a safe space.**

*What is a safe space?*

### <u>SAFE SPACE DEFINITION</u>

*A Safe Space is a Judgment-Free Zone*

*In other words…*

*A safe space is:*
*A space where you can express yourself without attack*
*A space that has been prepared for you to enter into it*
*However you are in the moment.*

*Who is the safe space for?*

The safe space is first for you.
When you have created a safe space for yourself,
You can extend it to your Partner.

*How do you create a safe space?*

A safe space is first created in **your mind,**
By setting your intention.

> ## <u>INTENTION DEFINITION</u>
> ### *An "Intention" is an "Undivided Decision"*

## EXAMPLE OF SETTING YOUR INTENTION

When you set the intention for a "judgment-free zone"
You are making the undivided decision that:

### *"I Will Not Judge Anything That Happens Here"*

*Back to creating a safe space.*

**To create a safe space for yourself,
You must set the intention that you will:**

- *Be open with yourself*

- *Be honest with yourself*

- *Be genuine and gentle with yourself*

**To create a safe space for your Partner,
You must set the intention that you will:**

- *Be open with your Partner*

- *Be interested in what they have to share*

- *Be supportive and nurturing to them
No matter what comes up for them*

Now let's talk about how to do this.

# FINDING YOUR TOTEM
## *For Your Safe Space*

Even though the safe space is created internally by your intention,
It is helpful to have something external and physical
To represent that intention.

We will call this external thing a **TOTEM.**

### *What is a totem?*

## <u>TOTEM DEFINITION</u>
*Any Object That You Give the Following Meaning to:*
*"It Is Now A Safe Space For Us To Communicate Freely"*

You need a Totem to represent your safe space.

### *What are some examples of totems?*

## TOTEM EXAMPLES

- **A candle that you burn when you are together**
  - *When the candle is lit it means:*
    - *"This is now a safe space for us to communicate freely"*
- **A picture or quote that you put up on your wall or table**
  - *It could be as simple as a sticky note that says: "this is a safe space now"*
- **An item of clothing**
  - *Shirt, pants, socks, scarf, belt, etc*
    - *When you wear it, it means: "this is a safe space"*

- **A piece of jewelry**
  - *Bracelet, ring, necklace, earings*
    - *You can put it on each other to indicate "this is a safe space"*
- **A specific meal or snack**
  - *Bowl of fruit, chips, etc*
    - *When you are sharing this meal it means: "this is a safe space for use to communicate"*
- **A book, such as: "Beyond 50 Shades: *A Guide for Healthy Sexual Communication*"**
  - *You can decide together that whenever you bring out this Guide it means:*
    - *"This is a safe space for us to communicate about sex"*

You and your Partner have to decide what your totem will be.
Have a conversation and exchange ideas.

**What does it mean when the Totem is present?**

When you bring out your Totem, it means that now it is time
To do sexual communication healing work.
And this object (totem) means that
**"It is safe for us to communicate freely and openly about sex".**

If you haven't discussed and chosen a Totem yet,
Now is the time to do so.
Please have the conversation now,
And do not continue reading until you have chosen a Totem.

Ask your Partner this question:
**"What do you think our Totem should be?"**

**Go!**

# <u>SAFE SPACE RULES</u>

## *Remember These Rules*

**Here are some rules for your safe space:**

- **TURN OFF YOUR PHONES AND LEAVE THEM OUTSIDE OF THE ROOM!**
- **Schedule time for this just like you would an important meeting**
- **Prepare in advance by writing down questions that you are curious about**
- **Allow anything to come up emotionally for both of you**
  - *Laughter, tears, joy, fears*
- **When a block or past trauma comes up for your Partner around something, do not offer unsolicited advice or try to "fix" them**
  - *There is nothing wrong with them. Encountering blocks are part of the process*
- **Do not abandon the space or the conversation when it gets difficult or you feel triggered**
  - *State how you feel and sit with that feeling*
  - *If you want support from your Partner in any form, request help; ask them to hold space for you*
    - *Don't **expect** it*
    - *They don't owe you any form of support*
    - *Appreciate any support they offer as a gift*
- **Take responsibility for your feelings, your blocks, your hangups, and your hurt**
  - *Do not place the responsibility for your feelings on your Partner*
    - *Remember this: If they did not physically harm you, they did nothing to you*
      - *It is impossible for someone to "hurt" you emotionally - you did it to yourself*

## <u>SAFE SPACE RULES</u> (continued)

- **If you don't want to talk about something, don't talk about it**
  - *A safe space is not a space to "tell all"*
    - *There are probably some things you don't want to share with anyone, and you don't have to*
  - *A safe space is a space to "**share what you want to share without fear or attack**"*
- **Do not pressure your Partner to talk, share, respond or answer any of your questions**
  - *A safe space means you are safe NOT to talk also*
- **Encourage and appreciate each other throughout the process**

---

# APPRECIATE EACH OTHER
### *End Every Session With Appreciation*

Sexual healing work is not always easy,
But it is necessary if you want healthy sexual communication.
You deserve to be appreciated for
The healing work you are doing together.

***And who do you think is going to***
***Appreciate you and your Partner for the work you're doing?***

### YOU ARE!

Which is why now you're going to learn and practice an exercise
That will help you easily express appreciation to each other.

*Ready?*

**Please continue.**

# APPRECIATION EXERCISE
### *Three Simple Questions*

## PURPOSE OF THIS EXERCISE

The purpose of this exercise and practice is to remind yourself
And your Partner of the appreciation you have for each other.

### Starting with yourself first.

By doing this healing work together you are saving yourselves
*Years* of future pain, trauma, and frustrating
Sexual and communication blocks.

After every session you spend together in your safe space,
End the session by asking each other
The following three questions:

---

## APPRECIATION EXERCISE QUESTIONS
### *Aim for 1-3 answers for each question*

*What is something you appreciate about yourself?*

*What is something you appreciate about me?*

*What is something you appreciate about our relationship?*

---

### That's it!

What we are giving you are the basic foundational tools for
Healthy sexual communication.

If you USE these tools consistently,
You will find your comfort and peace around
Sexuality in your life and relationships blossom.

You can expand on this exercise by asking related questions.

**FOR EXAMPLE**

## RELATED APPRECIATION QUESTIONS

*What is something you appreciated about our session?*
*What is something you learned about me in our session?*
*What is something you learned about yourself in our session?*

Have fun, and don't walk away from a session
Or from your safe space without doing the
**APPRECIATION EXERCISE.**

---

Now let's bring it home.

# CONCLUSION
*Cheat Codes!*

Let's conclude this Chapter with some Cheat Codes on the
Purpose of a safe space.

[See Cheat Codes Chart on Next Page]

# CHEAT CODES ON WHAT A SAFE SPACE IS FOR AND IS NOT FOR

| A SAFE SPACE IS NOT FOR | A SAFE SPACE IS FOR |
|---|---|
| *Arguments* | *Sharing freely* |
| *Attack* | *Appreciation* |
| *Going back and forth with each other* | *Listening attentively and actively* |
| *Being distracted* | *Giving your full attention* |
| *Trying to change your Partner or getting them to do something differently* | *Learning more about your Partner and accepting them exactly as they are* |
| *Changing something about yourself* | *Accepting yourself exactly as you are* |
| *Voicing disgust, disapproval or judgment about your Partner* | *Voicing appreciation or being silent* |
| *Avoiding emotional discomfort Avoiding feeling triggered Shutting down to your Partner When you feel triggered* | *Feeling triggered, sitting with that feeling and knowing that you are safe even if you're feeling emotionally uncomfortable in the moment* |
| *Discussing things you find easy and comfortable talking about and asking your Partner about* | *Discussing things that are uncomfortable and difficult for you to talk about and ask your Partner about* |

*Clear?*

**Moving on!**

# Part II

# SEXPLORATION

*Sexual Communication Topics*

### Let's Talk About Sex!

In this part, we will explore different topics related to sex.

### Why?

So you and your Partner can communicate about it.

Before we begin, there are two rules you must both agree to.

# RULES FOR SEXPLORATION
### 2 Rules

If you are adult enough to open to this section in this Guide,
You must be adult enough to follow these rules together.

### RULE #1
*No Judgment!*

This is a judgment-free zone.
Prepare your safe space before going into the conversations
To remind yourselves that this is a judgment-free zone.

### RULE #2
*No Pressure!*

If you don't want to answer any question...

*Guess what?*

**YOU DON'T HAVE TO ANSWER IT!**

And if your Partner doesn't want to answer any question...

*Guess what?*

**THEY DON'T HAVE TO ANSWER IT EITHER!**

You don't have to do anything you don't want to do.

When in doubt, review rules 1 and 2.

**NO JUDGMENT! NO PRESSURE!**

*Ready to explore your sexuality?*

**Turn the page!**

# <u>Chapter 5</u>
# SEX?
### *Let's Talk About Sex*

Let's start simple.

Here you're going to have a discussion
With your Partner about sex.
Follow the instructions.

## INSTRUCTIONS

1) Start by creating/setting up your safe space

2) When you are settled, turn to the next page and use
   the questions to Guide your conversation about sex

## NOTE
*To help better gauge where you are with certain questions,*
*You can use a number scale of 0 - 10 to communicate your answer.*

*"0" meaning "nothing", "not important" or "no experience in that area"*
*"10" being "everything", "extremely important" or*
*"A lot experience in that area"*

3) Remember this is a safe space, so you don't have to answer
   any questions you don't want to answer

Take your time.
Ask each other the same question if it applies.
You don't have to go through the whole list in one session.

*And most importantly...*

**Have fun!**

# QUESTIONS ABOUT SEX
## *Use These Questions To Guide Your Conversation And Deepen Your Sexual Communication*
### *(No particular order)*

*What does sex mean to you?*

*What do you ultimately want to experience by having sex?*

*Are you a virgin?*

*How old were you when you had your first sexual experience?*

*What was your first sexual experience like?*

*How would you define your sexual expression at this time in your life?*
*(Heterosexual, homosexual, bisexual, pansexual, sexually fluid, asexual, etc.)*

*What is your definition of intimacy?*

*How important is sex in a romantic relationship to you? 0-10*

*How important is intimacy to you before/during/after sex? 0-10*

*How skillful would you say you are at sex? 0-10*

*Do you think you would be happy in our relationship with no sex? Why? Or why not?*

*What do you want to explore sexually with me?*
*What do you want to improve or learn more about sexually?*

*Do you masturbate/self-pleasure?*

*What are some of your favorite sexual activities?*

*What is your favorite sex position(s)?*

*Where do you want to have sex?*

# QUESTIONS ABOUT SEX (continued)
## *Use These Questions To Guide Your Conversation And Deepen Your Sexual Communication*

*What turns you on the most about sex?*

*Have you ever practiced celibacy? Why?*

*Do you plan to practice celibacy? Why or why not?*

*How do you like to be approached before sex?*

*Do you like rough sex? How rough? Why or why not?*

*Do you want hold each other or to be held after sex?*

*How do you like to be touched? What are your sweet spots?*

*How important is orgasm to you durning sex? 0-10*

*How important is ejaculation to you during sex? 0-10*

*How important is it to you that I orgasm during sex? 0-10*

*How important is it to you that I ejaculate during sex? 0-10*

*How can I tell when you're having an orgasm?*

*Will you let me know if I'm doing something you don't like?*

*How long is your ideal sexual session?*

*How important is the length of our sexual sessions?*

*Do you like quickies?*

*How important is size (endowment) to you 0-10?*

Now that we talked about the fun stuff,
It's time to talk about some important sexual matters.

**Sexual Health and Safety.**

*Safe Space Ready?*

**Turn the page.**

# Chapter 6

# SEXUAL HEALTH?

## *Practicing Safe Sex*

### SCENARIO

Two Partners are reading this book together
*(Which happens to be their safe space totem)*
And they turn to this chapter on "sexual health".

### PARTNER 1

*Do you want to talk about sexual health?*

### PARTNER 2

*Yes. Let's!*

### PARTNER 1

*Ok. Question #1:*
*"How do you take care of your sexual health?"*

### PARTNER 2

*I get tested 2 weeks before my birthday every year.*
*When the results come in, it's like a birthday gift to myself.*

### PARTNER 1

*That's a great practice.*
*Your birthday's coming up soon, would you like to get tested together?*

### PARTNER 2

*I would!*
*How's next Wednesday work for you?*

### PARTNER 1

*I'll put it on my calendar right now.*
[Pause]

*Guess what?*

It's time to talk about sexual health!

*Ready?*

**Let's begin.**

---

## FIRST THINGS FIRST!

Set up your safe space.
When you have settled into your safe space together,
Continue reading and have this conversation.

Here are some questions to ask each other about sexual health.

# SEXUAL HEALTH CONVERSATION QUESTIONS

*Note: There are questions that are clearly directed at specific genders and body parts*
*If the question doesn't apply to you, it doesn't apply.*
*Use your common sense*

*How do you take care of your sexual health?*

*On a scale of 0-10,*
*How confident are you about your sexual health practices?*

*When is the last time you were tested for STIs*
*(Sexually Transmitted Infection)?*
*What were the results?*

*When is the last time you were tested for HIV?*
*What were the results?*

# SEXUAL HEALTH CONVERSATION QUESTIONS
### Continued...

*When do you plan to get tested again?*

*How often should we agree to get tested?*
*(Every 12-months? Every 6-months? Every 3 months?)*

*Would you like to get tested together sometime?*

If so, set a date RIGHT NOW

---

*Are you open to using birth-control methods when we have sex?*
*What kinds?*

### <u>EXAMPLES</u>
Condoms, birth control rings/patches,
contraceptive injection, IUD, sterilization,
Emergency contraceptive (morning after pill), etc.

*Do you want to use condoms when having sex? What kinds?*

*Do you want children?*

*Do you want children with me?*

*Do you want to have barrier-free (unprotected) sex with me?*

*What would you want to do if our sex resulted in pregnancy?*

*Have you ever had an STI?*

*If you have other sexual Partners,*
*do you practice birth control with them?*

*What methods of birth control do you use*
*with other sexual Partners?*

# SEXUAL HEALTH CONVERSATION QUESTIONS
### Continued...

*Have you ever taken a sexual health class
or watched a sexual education video? What did you learn?*

*Would you like to take a course
Or watch a sexual education video together?
(You can pull one up online for free)*

*Do you have any suggestions for how we can better protect
and take care of our sexual health?*

*What are some dealbreakers for you when it comes to sex?*

*In other words... Complete this sentence:*

*"I will not have sex with you if*

_______________________________________ *"*

*Good talk right?*

Now, onto our next topic!

**Sexual Identity.**

Let's gain some clarity on how you identify sexually.

*Ready?*

**Please continue.**

# Chapter 7
# SEXUAL IDENTITY?
### *Explore...Question...Discover*

Your sexual identity is not limited to your gender or your past.
Like you, your sexual identity is always evolving and growing,
And may be difficult to put into words.

***Even so,***
In your sexual communication journey,
This is an important area of clarity and communication.

Use the following questions to have a conversation
About your sexual identity.

Use these general questions to communicate and uncover
Deeper curiosity about your and your Partner's sexual expression.

**Questions to ask each other:**

*How do you identify your gender?*

- *Male*
- *Female*

- *Transgender*
- _______________

*How do you prefer to be addressed?*

- *Him/He*
- *Her/She*

- *They/Them*
- _______________

## Do You Have/Claim A Sexual Identity?
## If So, What is Your Sexual Identity?

- Heterosexual/Straight
- Homosexual/Gay
- Queer
- Bisexual
- Pansexual

- Sapiosexual
- Sexually fluid
- Asexual
- Demisexual
- ___________________

*(Circle all the apply)*

---

# SEXUAL IDENTITY CONVERSATION QUESTION

*Are you sexually attracted to your gender?*
*Are you attracted to the opposite gender?*
*Are you attracted to both genders?*

*How has your sexual identity evolved*
*over the course of your life?*

*Anything else you would like to add*
*or discuss about sexual identity right now?*

*Anything else you think I should know*
*About your sexuality or sexual identity?*

---

***End Session With Appreciation Exercise***

# Chapter 8
# SEXUAL EXCLUSIVITY?
## *Monogamy and Nonmonogamy*

### SCENARIO
Two Partners sitting on their mat (their safe space totem)
And having a sexual communication session.

### PARTNER 1
*There's something I want to tell you*

### PARTNER 2
*Ok. I'm listening*

### PARTNER 1
*I've been sexually exclusive with you since we started having sex.
I haven't asked you if you've been having sex with other people,
and you don't have to tell me.
I know we never spoke about our relationship being exclusive or open...
It kind of just happened that way.*

### PARTNER 2
*I know...I've been kinda afraid of having this conversation.*

### PARTNER 1
*Me too. I didn't want it to ruin what we have.
Which is why I'm glad we're having it now.*

### PARTNER 2
*So, are you happy being sexually exclusive with me,
Or do you want us to have an open relationship?*

**PARTNER 1**

*For me, it's more about feeling free than it is about sex.*
*I just want to feel free to connect with whoever I want, however I want*
*without feeling like it will threaten what we have.*
*Or like you're going to feel threatened by someone else I connect with.*
*I don't know...How do you feel about that?*

**PARTNER 2**

*I feel the same way. What we have belongs to us.*
*No other relationship can change that or threaten that...*
*I've had past Partners try to control and limit me out of their own fear*
*and insecurity. I won't do that to you.*

**PARTNER 1**

*Thank you for making it easy to talk to you about this.*

**PARTNER 2**

*Thank you for bringing it up.*

**PARTNER 1**

*I'm glad we created a safe space to discuss it in.*

**PARTNER 2**

[Looks at the mat and touches it]
*Hmmm...Does that mean that as long as I have this mat with me*
*it's ok to stalk you?*

[Both laugh. Pause]

---

## VERY IMPORTANT!!!

The "sexual exclusivity" conversation is a conversation that
**MUST HAPPEN**
In any romantic or sexual relationship you are in.

*Why?*

Because more than likely, you live in a culture that promotes
And *assumes* **monogamy** (sexual exclusivity).
*Meaning...*
Monogamy is usually assumed between sexual and romantic
Partners even without them directly asking about it or stating it.

Further, the conversation about sexual exclusivity will usually
Erupt from a place of fear, insecurity and suspicion of
A Partner being "unfaithful".

**FYI**
That is *THE MOST <u>DANGEROUS</u> TIME*
To have that conversation!
**Ever.**

In a culture that sends contradictory and confusing messages
Such as this, one must ask:

*"If the topic of sexual exclusivity is so important,
Why is it not discussed very early on in relationships?"*

*Again...*
**Because sexual exclusivity is assumed.**

**<u>FALSE SEXUAL EXCLUSIVITY ASSUMPTION</u>**
*If We Don't Discuss or Say Otherwise,
We Are In a Monogamous (Sexually Exclusive) Relationship*

This is why it is so important that you have this conversation.
And have it many times...

*Why?*

**Because people change, values change, minds change,
Feelings change, attraction changes, circumstances change.**

You are not the same person you were 6 months ago.
And the person you are with is not the same person they were
6 months ago...
Even if you were together for 60 years.

**People change everyday.**

**Best to treat them like you're meeting them for the first time...**

*Every time.*

That said,
It's time to have the "sexual exclusivity" conversation.

Before proceeding, prepare your safe space and enter it together.

*Ready?*

**Let's begin.**

---

Here are some questions to ask each other
About sexual exclusivity.

Have this conversation now.

[Sexual Exclusivity Conversation Questions on next page]

# SEXUAL EXCLUSIVITY CONVERSATION QUESTIONS

*Does our relationship have a label/title?*

*If it doesn't, do you want it to have a label/title?*

*What does that label/title mean to you?*

*What does that label/title mean to you in terms of our sexual openness?*

*What does monogamy mean to you?*

*Do you want our sexual relations to be exclusive (monogamous)?*

*Do you prefer monogamy? Why? Why not?*

*What does non-monogamy mean to you?*

*Do you want our sexual relations to be nonexclusive (non-monogamous)?*

*Do you prefer non-monogamy? Why?*

*Would it bother you if I choose to remain sexually exclusive and you don't?*

*If I choose to have other sexual Partners, do you want to know?*

*Why?*

*Do you want to know how many? Why?*

*Do you believe what I do with other people sexually is any of your business? Why?*

*What are your personal boundaries around sexual Partners?*

*What boundaries would you feel comfortable setting for our sexual relationship?*

## SEXUAL EXCLUSIVITY CONVERSATION QUESTIONS (Continued)

*What is a deal-breaker situation for you?*

(Meaning, a situation where you no longer choose to have a
sexual relationship with me
Or anyone you're having sex with)

*Would you be open to discussing this again sometime?*

IMPORTANT!

***End session with your Appreciation Exercise***

Now that you've covered that important topic,
It's time to get it on!!!

*Or is it?*

*Wouldn't it be nice to know if and when your Partner
Is ready and willing to have sex with you?*

Not only is it nice…

*It's legally required.*

So let's talk about the *most important* <u>**safe word**</u> of them all…

*What word is that?*

**CONSENT!!!**

*Do you want to continue?????*

# Chapter 9

# CONSENT?

*How To Ask For It, How To Give it*

## SCENARIO

PARTNER 1 and PARTNER 2 are on a walk in the park at night.

## PARTNER 1

*Are you wearing underwear?*

## PARTNER 2

*No.*

## PARTNER 1

*[Leads PARTNER 2 to a secluded area]*

**[The next morning, both Partners are in bed]**

## PARTNER 1

*Sex was amazing last night. Such a thrill!*

## PARTNER 2

*Yeah! I didn't know how I would feel about sex outdoors…*
*I'm glad you didn't give me time to think too hard and psych myself out*

## PARTNER 1

*I remember what no underwear means…It was your idea after all…*

## PARTNER 2

*[Blushes]*
*It means you can fuck me anywhere, anytime…*
*Unless I say otherwise*

# PARTNER 1

[Looks up and down Partner 1's naked body…]
*Looks like you still never found any to put on…So does that mean…?*

# PARTNER 2

[Dramatically lays open and spread eagle on the bed]

[Both laugh.
Pause.]

---

The importance of consent in a sexual relationship is something
That cannot be stressed enough.

*Ready to talk about it?*

**Let's begin.**

---

*What is consent?*

## <u>DEFINITION OF CONSENT</u>
### *A Clear Unequivocal Agreement To Engage In Sexual Activity*

To be very clear, let's ask and answer the big questions regarding
consent:

*Who must you gain consent from?*

Whomever you are engaging in sexual activity with.

*When must consent be gained?*

**Before every sexual act.**
**Each and every time.**

*"What if we have sex frequently?*
*Do I still have to ask for consent every time?*
*Do I still have to grant consent every time?"*

**Absolutely.**

*EVERY*　　　　*DAMN*　　　　*TIME.*

**It doesn't matter if you're married and on your honeymoon.**

## <u>CONSENT PRINCIPLE</u>
*Yesterday's Consent Means Absolutely Nothing Today*
*Ask Every Time*

*When can consent be revoked?*

**Consent can be revoked at any point**
**Before or during sexual activity.**

*When can consent NOT be given?*

**IMPORTANT!!!**

*Consent Can NOT be given by someone who is...*
- **Under the legal age of an adult**
- **Under the influence of drugs or alcohol**
- **Forced, coerced or threatened into agreeing to sex**
- **Sleeping or unconscious**

In those cases, even if the person enthusiastically says:

*"Yes! Yes! Yes! I want you to fuck me! Right now!!! Yes!!!"*

It still does not count as consent. And if you have sex with them,
They can file criminal charges against you.

*Why?*

Because you just committed a crime against them
**It's called "sexual assault".**

Yes, even if you're happily married to them.
**It's still sexual assault.**

*Why are we going over consent?*

Because it is essential.
And unfortunately it is thought of as being *implied*
Especially in sexually active relationships.

**Let's get one thing straight right now.**

## <u>CONSENT PRINCIPLE</u>
*Consent should never be "implied"*
*Or believed to be implied*
*WITH ANYONE*
*EVER*

*Why?*

Because "implications" and "beliefs" are not certainties.
**They are suspect.**

Consent is not something you can "suspect" or roll the dice on.

Consent is **essential** for a healthy sexual relationship,
And a topic that cannot be overcommunicated.

*"So how do we do it?*
*How do we give, receive and discuss consent?"*

Time for your consent conversation!

*Do you consent to having this conversation?*

---

# CLARIFYING CONSENT CONVERSATION QUESTIONS

*How should we communicate about consent? Ideas?*

*Is there a specific way you like to be asked for consent?*

*Is there an approach you dislike?*

*Will you let me know when you want to have sex? How?*

*If one of us wants sex and the other doesn't at that time,*
*Can we make that ok?*
*And not to take it personally or see it as a shut-down or rejection?*

*Do you have any discomfort or hesitation when it comes to*
*approaching me about sex?*
*If so, why? Can you say where it's coming from?*

*How can we help each other minimize any pressure or discomfort*
*that comes up about it?*

---

---

# CLARIFYING CONSENT
# CONVERSATION QUESTIONS
### (Continued)

*Do you feel comfortable NOT AGREEING to sex with me?*

*If we have established consent for our sexual session
and you change your mind at any time,
will you let me know immediately?*

*How can we get fun and creative about consent?*

---

# CONSENT IS NOT ALWAYS VERBAL
## *Creative Consent Symbols*

Now that you've *verbally* articulated your thoughts
And agreements about consent,
### *Let's get creative!*

As you know, consent must be given before *EVERY* sexual act,
In *EVERY* sexual relationship.

*At the same time,*
You don't have to approach consent the same way every time.

*"So how can we communicate consent if we don't verbalize it?*

*How do I let my Partner know that I want to get it on
Without using words?"*

Easy.
**Create your own "consent" language between you two.**

*How?*

*By using symbols and getting creative.*

Check out the following Cheat Codes Chart
On Creating Consent Symbols.

## <u>NOTE</u>
*You don't have to use the examples listed,*
*They are just suggestions to give you some ideas.*
*You **DO** need to have a conversation with your Partner about*
*What symbols you both agree on though.*

## CREATING CONSENT SYMBOLS CHART
*Suggestions For Communicating Consent*

| CONSENT SYMBOL<br>Or Action | EXAMPLES<br>*This Means:*<br>*"I'm A Total Yes To Sex With You Right Now"* |
|---|---|
| Music | *When you play a certain song, artist,*<br>*Band or playlist* |
| Clothing<br>No Clothing | *When you wear a certain outfit, lingerie, etc*<br>*When you're totally naked* |
| Props, Items<br>Toys | *When certain items are brought out and placed*<br>*in a certain location*<br>*They don't necessarily have to be sexual items* |

### EXAMPLES
| | |
|---|---|
| *Leaving a condom on the pillow* | *Dimming the bedroom lights* |
| *Lighting a candle* | *Having sex toys on the bed* |
| *Porn Playing on the TV/Computer* | *Your Erotic Journal on the bed* |

| CREATING CONSENT SYMBOLS CHART | |
| --- | --- |
| *Suggestions For Communicating Consent (Continued)* | |
| **CONSENT SYMBOL** <br> *Or Action* | **EXAMPLES** <br> *This Means:* <br> *"I'm A Total Yes To Sex With You Right Now"* |
| **Written notes, Text Messages, etc** | *Leaving a note that expresses exactly how sexually frisky you're feeling* <br> *And what you want to do when you see your Partner later* <br> *Sending a text message to that effect* |
| **Physical Position** | *When you are in a certain position,* <br> *It means you're ready for sex* |
| **POSITION EXAMPLES** <br> **ON THE BED** <br> *Spread eagle, actively pleasuring yourself, face down ass in the air* | |
| **Bedding** | *When you make up the bed with a certain kind of [black satin] sheets or pillowcases* |
| **Lighting** | *When the lights are turned off of dim* |

Again, these are just suggestions to get your
Sexual minds lubricated.

Create your own symbols for consent.

*Ready to create something together?*

Have the conversation.

And do not go to the next chapter until
You have agreed on an answer to this question:

## CONVERSATION QUESTION
***"What is something we can use to mean
'I'm open and ready for sex'"?***

Talk about it!

**Now.**

---

In our next chapter,
We will explore how you like to get turned on before getting it on.

*What are we talking about now?*

## FOREPLAY

*Ready to play?*

**Turn the page.**

# Chapter 10
# FOREPLAY?
*Let's Talk About It!*

## SCENARIO
*Two Partners are in their safe space holding a conversation.*

## PARTNER 1
*How do you like to foreplay?*

## PARTNER 2
*I like it when we text throughout the day about about our fantasies,
and when you send me explicit pictures
By the time we see each other, I'm ready to jump on you!*

[Pause]

Time to talk about foreplay!

*Ready?*

**Let's begin.**

---

# COMMUNICATING ABOUT FOREPLAY
*Questions for Conversation*

Use the following questions to learn more about your Partner.

[Use the conversation Guide on the next page]

# FOREPLAY
# CONVERSATION QUESTIONS

*What is foreplay to you?*
*What does it mean to "foreplay" to you?*

*How do you like to foreplay?*
*What are some of your favorite ways to foreplay?*

*What is something you've never done that you're open to trying?*

*On a scale of 0-10,*
*0 being "unnecessary" and 10 being "extremely important"*
*How important is foreplay to you?*

Have the conversation now.

***END WITH APPRECIATION PRACTICE***

# Chapter 11
# TURN ONS AND TURN OFFS
### *Let's Talk About It!*

## PARTNER 1
*What are some of your turn ons?*

## PARTNER 2
*As a sapiosexual, I like when we have deep conversations
and I learn something new about you.
Discovering more and more ways to connect with you turns me on.*

[Pause]

---

Before we talk about your turn ons and turn offs,
Let's define the terms:

| |
|---|
| ### "TURN ON" DEFINITION<br>*Anything That Brings You Sensual and/or Sexual Pleasure* |

| |
|---|
| ### "TURN OFF" DEFINITION<br>*Anything That Does NOT Bring You Sensual<br>And/or Sexual Pleasure* |

Time to discuss your turn ons and turn offs!

*Safe Space Ready?*

**Let's begin.**

# COMMUNICATING ABOUT TURN ONS AND OFFS
### *Questions for Conversation*

Use the following questions to learn more about what
Turns each other on and off.

---

## QUESTIONS FOR COMMUNICATING ABOUT TURN ONS AND TURN OFFS

*What are some of your turn ons?*
*Name 3 of your biggest turn ons*

*What are some of your turn offs?*
*Name 3 of your biggest turn offs*

*What is something I do that turns you on?*
*What would you like (me/us) to do more of?*

---

In the following interactive Cheat Codes Chart,
You will be given a list of common
Sensual/erotic activities and a list of common sexual activities.

Next to each activity,
You can write/state how much it turns you on from 0-10.
A "0" being a "turn off" and "1-10"
Being the level you are turned on by the activity.

If you don't know how turned on you are by something,
Or if you've never tried it, use a question mark "?".

Use the blank spaces to fill in your own exotic/sexual activities at
the bottom of the lists.

## <u>NOTE ON TERMS</u>

*"Sensual/Erotic activities"*
*Are not necessarily <u>sexually</u> stimulating.*
*They can simply be arousing.*

*They can also be done during the course of a sexual session.*

*"Sexual activities" are intentionally sexually stimulating,*
*And are meant to be part of a sexual session.*

# CHEAT CODES CHART FOR *TURN ONS AND TURN OFFS*
### *"How Turned On Are Your By…?"*

| SENSUAL/ EROTIC ACTIVITY | TURNED ON 0-10? | SEXUAL ACTIVITY | TURNED ON 0-10? |
|---|---|---|---|
| Kissing | | Vaginal Sex | |
| Cuddling | | Oral Sex | |
| Dirty talk | | Anal Sex | |
| Sweet talk | | Using toys during sex | |
| Flirting | | Roleplay | |
| Seducing | | BDSM and Kink | |
| Foreplay | | Masturbation | |
| Spanking | | Mutual Masturbation | |
| Massage | | Orgasm denial | |

<table>
<tr><th colspan="4">CHEAT CODES CHART FOR<br>TURN ONS AND TURN OFFS<br>"How Turned On Are Your By…?"<br>(Continued)</th></tr>
<tr><th>SENSUAL/<br>EROTIC<br>ACTIVITY</th><th>TURNED<br>ON<br>0-10?</th><th>SEXUAL<br>ACTIVITY</th><th>TURNED<br>ON<br>0-10?</th></tr>
<tr><td>Dressing up/<br>Lingerie</td><td></td><td>Watching others<br>have sex</td><td></td></tr>
<tr><td>Blindfolds</td><td></td><td>Others watching<br>you have sex</td><td></td></tr>
<tr><td>Watching Porn</td><td></td><td>Outdoor sex</td><td></td></tr>
<tr><td>Being Tied Up</td><td></td><td>Group sex</td><td></td></tr>
<tr><td>Tying Up Partner</td><td></td><td>Making home sex tapes</td><td></td></tr>
<tr><td></td><td></td><td></td><td></td></tr>
<tr><td></td><td></td><td></td><td></td></tr>
<tr><td></td><td></td><td></td><td></td></tr>
</table>

*Are you ready to get spicy?*

**Let's talk about kinks and fetishes now!**

# Chapter 12
# KINKS AND FETISHES?
## *"Alternative" Sexual Practices*

## SCENARIO

Two Partners are browsing an adult store together.
They wander into the kinky section...

## PARTNER 1

[Pulls down a pair of handcuffs from the shelf]
*Have you ever been handcuffed?*

## PARTNER 2

*[Shakes head]*
*Not in the bedroom anyway.*
*[Both laugh]*
*Do you want to try it?*

## PARTNER 1

*Yeah, I would.*

## PARTNER 2

*What did you have in mind?*

## PARTNER 1

*I was thinking, let's use them in roleplay tonight.*
*You be an off-duty cop...*
*I'll be an escaped prisoner who breaks into your apartment...*

## PARTNER 2

*And you find my handcuffs while I'm sleeping...*

**PARTNER 1**

*Which I use to handcuff you to the bedpost,*
*and then have my way with you...all night long.*


**PARTNER 2**

*Promise?*


[Pause]

---

Now it's time to talk about the taboo stuff.

**"Kinks and fetishes"**

*In other words...*

### <u>KINK AND FETISH DEFINITION</u>
*Alternative or Unusual Sexual Practices*

*Ready?*

**Let's get kinky.**

---

# GETTING IN TOUCH
# WITH YOUR KINKY SIDE
*Kinky Conversation-Exploration Guide*

On the following page is a chart with two lists
Of common kinks and fetishes.

Use the chart as a questionnaire, and conversation piece.
There are two copies so you and your Partner
Can fill it out together.

## HOW TO FILL OUT THE KINKY GUIDE

Next to each kink/fetish is a column that asks the question:
*"(Are you) Into it?"*

You can circle **"Yes" "No" or "Open"** if you are open to trying it.

The next column asks:
*"Give / Receive / Both"*

Here you write the letter **"G"** for "give",
**"R"** for "receive", or **"B"** for "both".

This column doesn't qualify for some kinks and fetishes
Such as "watching porn together".
Use your discernment.

## WHAT IT TELLS YOU

Let's say for the "Sex Toys" kink/fetish, you circle "Yes",
And in the next column you write the letter **"B"**.

This means *"Yes"* you are into *"Both"* using sex toys on your
Partner, and having them use sex toys on you.

The details of that sexual exploration you will have to
Communicate with each other about.

*"What if I come across some terms I'm not familiar with?"*

That's a good sign.

86

It means you're expanding your sexual knowledge and horizons.

If you haven't heard of some of the kinks/fetishes on the list,
Or you are not sure what they are…

*Look it up!*

**That's what the internet is for.**

It might spark an interesting, eye-opening sexy conversation.
*You never know....*

*That's why you're doing this isn't it?*

**Now let's get to it.**

*[Two copies of "Kinky Conversation Exploration Guide"
On next pages]*

## KINKY CONVERSATION EXPLORATION GUIDE

(Partner 1 Name) _______________________________

| KINK/ FETISH *Detail* | Into it? | Give/ Receive /Both | KINK/ FETISH *Detail* | Into it? | Give/ Receive/ Both |
|---|---|---|---|---|---|
| **Impact Play** *Spanking, Paddling* | Yes/ No/ Open | | **Group Sex** *Threesomes, Swinging, etc* | Yes/ No/ Open | |
| **Bondage** *Binding with rope* | Yes/ No/ Open | | **Hosiery & Outfits** *Lingerie, Latex, etc* | Yes/ No/ Open | |
| **Sadism** *Inflicting Pain Brings pleasure* | Yes/ No/ Open | | **Home Movies** *Making your own sex tapes* | Yes/ No/ Open | |
| **Masochism** *Receiving Pain Brings pleasure* | Yes/ No/ Open | | **Forced Fantasies (CNC)** *"Consensual Non-Consent"* | Yes/ No/ Open | |
| **Sex Toys** *Using sex toys during sex* | Yes/ No/ Open | | **Voyeurism** *Watching Sexual Acts* | Yes/ No/ Open | |
| **Orgasm Control** *Forcing and/or Withholding Orgasms* | Yes/ No/ Open | | **Sensation/ Sensory Play** *Temperature play, heat, ice, Sensory deprivation* | Yes/ No/ Open | |
| **Age Playing** *Pretending to be a different age* | Yes/ No/ Open | | **Exhibitionism** *Having sex in front of others or in public* | Yes/ No/ Open | |

# KINKY CONVERSATION EXPLORATION GUIDE

(Partner 1 Name) _______________________________ (Continued)

| KINK/ FETISH<br>*Detail* | *Are You Into it?* | Give/ Receive /Both | KINK/ FETISH<br>*Detail* | *Are You Into it?* | Give/ Receive /Both |
|---|---|---|---|---|---|
| **Domination**<br>*Dominating* | *Yes/No /Open* | | **Going to Sex Parties** | *Yes/No/ Open* | |
| **Submission**<br>*Submitting* | *Yes/No /Open* | | **Going to Sex Dungeons** | *Yes/No/ Open* | |
| **Blindfolding** | *Yes/No /Open* | | **Going to Adult Stores** | *Yes/No/ Open* | |
| **Biting** | *Yes/No /Open* | | **Foot Fetish** | *Yes/No/ Open* | |
| **Nipple Play** | *Yes/No /Open* | | **Collaring** | *Yes/No/ Open* | |
| **Watersports** | *Yes/No /Open* | | **Pegging** | *Yes/No/ Open* | |
| **Wax Play** | *Yes/No /Open* | | **Cuckolding** | *Yes/No/ Open* | |
| **Role Playing** | *Yes/No /Open* | | **Electro-play** | *Yes/No/ Open* | |
| **Watch Porn Together** | *Yes/No /Open* | | **Whipping** | *Yes/No/ Open* | |
| **Gagging** | *Yes/No /Open* | | **Fingering/ Handjobs** | *Yes/No/ Open* | |

## KINKY CONVERSATION EXPLORATION GUIDE

(Partner 1 Name) ___________________________ (Continued)

| KINK/ FETISH *Detail* | *Are You Into it?* | Give/ Receive /Both | KINK/ FETISH *Detail* | *Are You Into it?* | Give/ Receive /Both |
|---|---|---|---|---|---|
| Handcuffs | Yes / No / Open | | Sensual Erotic Massage | Yes / No / Open | |
| Marks (Hickies) | Yes / No / Open | | Prostate Play | Yes / No / Open | |
| Consensual Non-Monogamy | Yes / No / Open | | Rough Play (*Hair Pulling, Face Slapping*) | Yes / No / Open | |
| Anal Sex | Yes / No / Open | | Dirty Talk/ Sweet Talk | Yes / No / Open | |
| Face sitting | Yes / No / Open | | Oral Sex | Yes / No / Open | |
| Paying for sex | Yes / No / Open | | Sexting | Yes / No / Open | |
| CBT | Yes / No / Open | | Straitjacket | Yes / No / Open | |
| Stripping Erotic Dance | Yes / No / Open | | Oils and Lotion | Yes / No / Open | |

# KINKY CONVERSATION EXPLORATION GUIDE

(Partner 2 Name) ________________________________

| KINK/ FETISH Detail | Into it? | Give/ Receive /Both | KINK/ FETISH Detail | Into it? | Give/ Receive/ Both |
|---|---|---|---|---|---|
| **Impact Play** *Spanking, Paddling* | Yes/ No/ Open | | **Group Sex** *Threesomes, Swinging, etc* | Yes/ No/ Open | |
| **Bondage** *Binding with rope* | Yes/ No/ Open | | **Hosiery & Outfits** *Lingerie, Latex, etc* | Yes/ No/ Open | |
| **Sadism** *Inflicting Pain Brings pleasure* | Yes/ No/ Open | | **Home Movies** *Making your own sex tapes* | Yes/ No/ Open | |
| **Masochism** *Receiving Pain Brings pleasure* | Yes/ No/ Open | | **Forced Fantasies (CNC)** *"Consensual Non-Consent"* | Yes/ No/ Open | |
| **Sex Toys** *Using sex toys during sex* | Yes/ No/ Open | | **Voyeurism** *Watching Sexual Acts* | Yes/ No/ Open | |
| **Orgasm Control** *Forcing and/or Withholding Orgasms* | Yes/ No/ Open | | **Sensation/ Sensory Play** *Temperature play, heat, ice, Sensory deprivation* | Yes/ No/ Open | |
| **Age Playing** *Pretending to be a different age* | Yes/ No/ Open | | **Exhibitionism** *Having sex in front of others or in public* | Yes/ No/ Open | |

# KINKY CONVERSATION EXPLORATION GUIDE

(Partner 2 Name) _________________________ (Continued)

| KINK/ FETISH *Detail* | *Are You* Into it? | Give/ Receive /Both | KINK/ FETISH *Detail* | *Are You* Into it? | Give/ Receive /Both |
|---|---|---|---|---|---|
| Domination *Dominating* | Yes/No /Open | | Going to Sex Parties | Yes/No/ Open | |
| Submission *Submitting* | Yes/No /Open | | Going to Sex Dungeons | Yes/No/ Open | |
| Blindfolding | Yes/No /Open | | Going to Adult Stores | Yes/No/ Open | |
| Biting | Yes/No /Open | | Foot Fetish | Yes/No/ Open | |
| Nipple Play | Yes/No /Open | | Collaring | Yes/No/ Open | |
| Watersports | Yes/No /Open | | Pegging | Yes/No/ Open | |
| Wax Play | Yes/No /Open | | Cuckolding | Yes/No/ Open | |
| Role Playing | Yes/No /Open | | Electro-play | Yes/No/ Open | |
| Watch Porn Together | Yes/No /Open | | Whipping | Yes/No/ Open | |
| Gagging | Yes/No /Open | | Fingering/ Handjobs | Yes/No/ Open | |

# KINKY CONVERSATION EXPLORATION GUIDE

(Partner 2 Name) ___________________________ (Continued)

| KINK/ FETISH *Detail* | *Are You Into it?* | Give/ Receive /Both | KINK/ FETISH *Detail* | *Are You Into it?* | Give/ Receive /Both |
|---|---|---|---|---|---|
| Handcuffs | Yes/No/ Open | | Sensual Erotic Massage | Yes/No/ Open | |
| Marks (Hickies) | Yes/No/ Open | | Prostate Play | Yes/No/ Open | |
| Consensual Non-Monogamy | Yes/No/ Open | | Rough Play (Hair Pulling, Face Slapping) | Yes/No/ Open | |
| Anal Sex | Yes/No/ Open | | Dirty Talk/ Sweet Talk | Yes/No/ Open | |
| Face sitting | Yes/No/ Open | | Oral Sex | Yes/No/ Open | |
| Paying for sex | Yes/No/ Open | | Sexting | Yes/No/ Open | |
| CBT | Yes/No/ Open | | Straitjacket | Yes/No/ Open | |
| Stripping Erotic Dance | Yes/No/ Open | | Oils and Lotion | Yes/No/ Open | |

***End With Appreciation Exercise***

# <u>Chapter 13</u>
# PORN?
### *What Do You Watch?*

## SCENARIO
*Two Partners are in their safe space holding a conversation.*

## PARTNER 1
*What kind of porn do you watch?*

## PARTNER 2
*I like hentai porn*

## PARTNER 1
[Confused look]
*What the hell is that?*

## PARTNER 2
[Pulls out laptop]
*Let me show you…*

[Pause]

Time to talk about porn!

### *Ready?*

**Let's begin.**

# COMMUNICATING ABOUT PORN
## *Questions for Conversation*

Use the following questions to learn more about your Partner

## PORNOGRAPHY
## CONVERSATION QUESTIONS

*Do you watch porn? Why? Why not?*

*What kinds of porn do you like? What turns you on about it?*

*Who are some of your favorite porn stars?*

*Have you ever considered doing porn?*

*Can you introduce me to some of your
favorite porn sites and videos?*

*Would you be open to watching some porn together?*

*Have you ever thought about shooting our own private sex film?*

*What do you want to do in it?*

Have the conversation now.

***END WITH APPRECIATION PRACTICE***

# Chapter 14
# EROTIC JOURNAL
### *Your Literary Safe Space*

*Do you want to bring your sexual communication
To the next level?*

For this final chapter,
We are going to offer a very simple and
Powerful tool that will help you do just that.

*What tool is that?*

**An erotic journal.**

*What is the purpose of an erotic journal?*

An erotic journal is another safe space to communicate freely
About sex with your Partner.

Sometimes, you may find it easier
To write about things than to talk about them.
This journal gives you another outlet to express yourself.

*What do you write about in your erotic journal?*

You can write about anything and everything
On your sexual mind.

**Such as:**

- *Your desires*
- *Your fantasies*
- *What you like*
- *What you want to explore*
- *What you want to do again*
- *What you learned*
- *Setting the goal exercise*

Now let's talk about what your erotic journal is and is not.

| YOUR EROTIC JOURNAL CHEAT CODES | |
| --- | --- |
| **YOUR EROTIC JOURNAL <u>IS NOT</u>** | **YOUR EROTIC JOURNAL <u>IS</u>** |
| **NOT PUBLIC**<br>*Not for anyone and everyone*<br>*to know about* | **PRIVATE**<br>*It is between you*<br>*and your Partner* |
| **NOT A PLACE TO ATTACK OR FEEL ATTACKED**<br>*Do not attack, criticize*<br>*or shame your Partner or yourself* | **A SAFE SPACE**<br>*A safe space to*<br>*communicate and connect*<br>*About your sexuality* |
| **NOT A ONE MAN SHOW**<br>*It's not for just one Partner*<br>*to write in all the time* | **FOR BOTH PARTNERS TO USE TOGETHER**<br>*Either use it together*<br>*or not at all* |

*Clear?*

Now it's time to have a conversation with your Partner.
This conversation consists of only one question.
Ask each other this question:

***"Do you want to start an erotic journal with me?"***

<u>**NOTE**</u>
*Answer that question before you continue reading*

# STARTING YOUR
# EROTIC JOURNAL TOGETHER
*Go Get The Book*

Once you and your Partner have decided that you want to
Start an erotic journal together,
Let's answer this question:

*"How do we start an erotic journal?"*

Follow these simple instructions:

## EROTIC JOURNAL INSTRUCTIONS

1. Get a blank notebook/journal from the store
2. Title it: ***Our Erotic Journal (or whatever name you want)***
3. Both of you write an entry in it! **IMMEDIATELY!!!**

If you are ever drawing a blank on what to write…
*Use the following "Erotic Journal Entry Guide"*

---

## EROTIC JOURNAL ENTRY GUIDE
*Use These Questions To Help Focus Your Entries*

*What do I appreciate about our
sexual communication and connection?
What do I appreciate about our sexual relationship?
What do I enjoy doing with you sexually?
What is something I want to do again?
What is a sexual block I have overcome or overcoming?
What fantasies do I want to explore with you?
What porn do I want to watch (or shoot) with you?
What roleplay scenarios do I want to play with?
What do I find sexy about you/us?
What have I discovered about myself (sexually) in our relationship?
What are some of the ways you turn me on?*

There are no rules for how long or articulate the entry has to be.

A valid entry can be one sentence, or a fun, sexy game you play...

## ENTRY EXAMPLE

*"Good day!*
*I would like to make an appointment with your nipples ASAP.*
*Please circle their availability*

- *Right now*

- *Tonight*

- *Tomorrow night*

- *Anytime you wish*

*I will reach out to them at my earliest convenience.*

*Sincerely,*

*-My tongue"*

---

There are no right or wrong, good or bad entries.
Just express yourself.

An erotic journal is of course an optional tool.
It is not required for healthy sexual communication.

But if you're going to commit to starting one together...
**USE IT!**

And most importantly,
*Have some damn fun.*

# *Congratulations!*

You have completed this Guide on:

## Beyond
*50 Shade*
*A Guide for Healthy Sexual Communication*

*So what do you have accomplished?*

By now, you should have accomplished the following...

You should have communicated thoroughly and clearly
About sex in your relationship.

You should have a healthy mindset about sex and sexuality.
You should have established a purpose for your relationship.

You should know how to hold space for each other.
You should have a safe space.

You should have asked your Partner questions
You should have learned more about each other.

You should have the tools needed to continue
Having a healthy sexual communication with each other.

*Now that you have what you've set out for...*

*It's up to you both to keep it cumming*

# ABOUT THE AUTHOR

*My name is Na'Im Ansar Najieb.*

*I am here only to be Truly Helpful.*

*To know me is to know my name.*

**Na'Im** *means* **Blessings**
**Ansar** *means* **Helpful**
**Najieb** *means* **Excellence**

*My goal is to* **Bless** *the world by being* **Helpful** *in an* **Excellent** *way.*

*That is who I am.*

*Supporting you in your practice of nurturing healthy relationships*
*Is one of the ways I live up to my name to be Truly Helpful.*

*Thank you for reading!*

*[For more information, see the following page]*

# CONTACT INFORMATION

## *For the Author, the Team and Relationship Support*

Na'Im and his team consults and conducts hands-on workshops
And seminars on:

> ### *How to Create and Maintain Healthy Relationships*

We believe that **Trust, Love and Communication (TLC)** are at the root of
**ALL HEALTHY RELATIONSHIPS.**

We specialize in *rapid and systematic healing* of troubled relationships.
As well as *maintaining and improving* Healthy Relationships.

We offer practical tools and training for all people
**No matter the type of relationship.**

---

**Do You Need Help With:**

*Improving your Family relationship dynamics?*
*Strained business and workplace relations?*
*Healing Heartbreak and Healthy Romantic Relationships?*
*Having Fulfilling Friendships and a Great Social Life?*
*Networking and Connecting with People Easily?*
*Team Building for Your Group or Company?*
*Improving Your Relationship with Yourself?*

**We Can Help!**

---

To Inquire about Booking, Private Clarity Sessions, Workshops, Appearances,
Events, Relationship Tools, Publications and more:

*Contact the Author!*
Naim@NaimNajieb.com

*Visit the Author!*
NaimNajieb.com